SPORTS IN THE NEWS

CONCUSSIONS

by Martin Gitlin

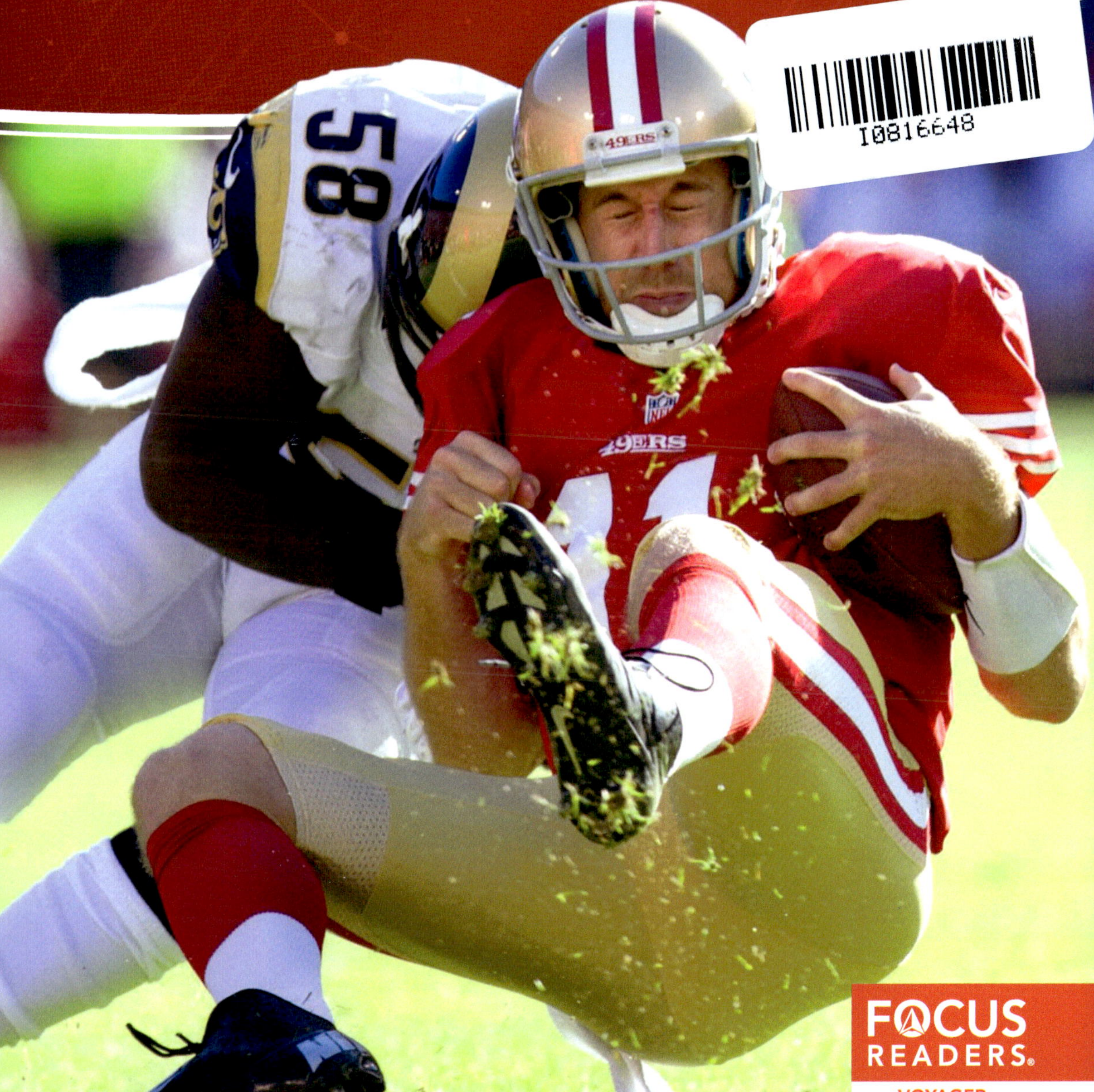

FOCUS READERS

VOYAGER

www.focusreaders.com

Focus Readers is distributed by North Star Editions:
sales@northstareditions.com | 888-417-0195

Produced for Focus Readers by Red Line Editorial.

Photographs ©: Paul Kitagaki Jr./The Sacramento Bee/AP Images, cover, 1; Charles Krupa/AP Images, 4–5; Shutterstock Images, 7, 11, 28–29, 33, 39, 42–43; David Durochik/AP Images, 8–9; Gene J. Puskar/AP Images, 13; Steven Senne/AP Images, 14–15; Greg Trott/AP Images, 17; Red Line Editorial, 19, 31; Ben Margot/AP Images, 21; Jeff Roberson/AP Images, 22–23; Kostas Lymperopoulos/Cal Sport Media/AP Images, 25; Morry Gash/AP Images, 27; Ryan Kang/AP Images, 34–35; Michael Ainsworth/AP Images, 37; Lloyd Fox/Baltimore Sun/TNS/Newscom, 41; Ron Waite/Cal Sport Media/AP Images, 45

Library of Congress Cataloging-in-Publication Data
Names: Gitlin, Marty, author.
Title: Concussions / by Martin Gitlin.
Description: Lake Elmo, MN : Focus Readers, [2021] | Series: Sports in the news | Includes index. | Audience: Grades 4-6
Identifiers: LCCN 2020005933 (print) | LCCN 2020005934 (ebook) | ISBN 9781644933916 (hardcover) | ISBN 9781644934678 (paperback) | ISBN 9781644936191 (pdf) | ISBN 9781644935439 (ebook)
Subjects: LCSH: Brain--Concussion--Juvenile literature. | Sports injuries--Juvenile literature.
Classification: LCC RC394.C7 G58 2021 (print) | LCC RC394.C7 (ebook) | DDC 617.4/81044--dc23
LC record available at https://lccn.loc.gov/2020005933
LC ebook record available at https://lccn.loc.gov/2020005934

Printed in the United States of America
Mankato, MN
082020

ABOUT THE AUTHOR

Martin Gitlin is an educational book author based in Cleveland, Ohio. He won more than 45 awards as a newspaper sportswriter from 1991 to 2002, including first place for general excellence from the Associated Press. That organization also voted him as one of the top four feature writers in Ohio. Gitlin has had more than 150 educational and trade books published since 2006.

TABLE OF CONTENTS

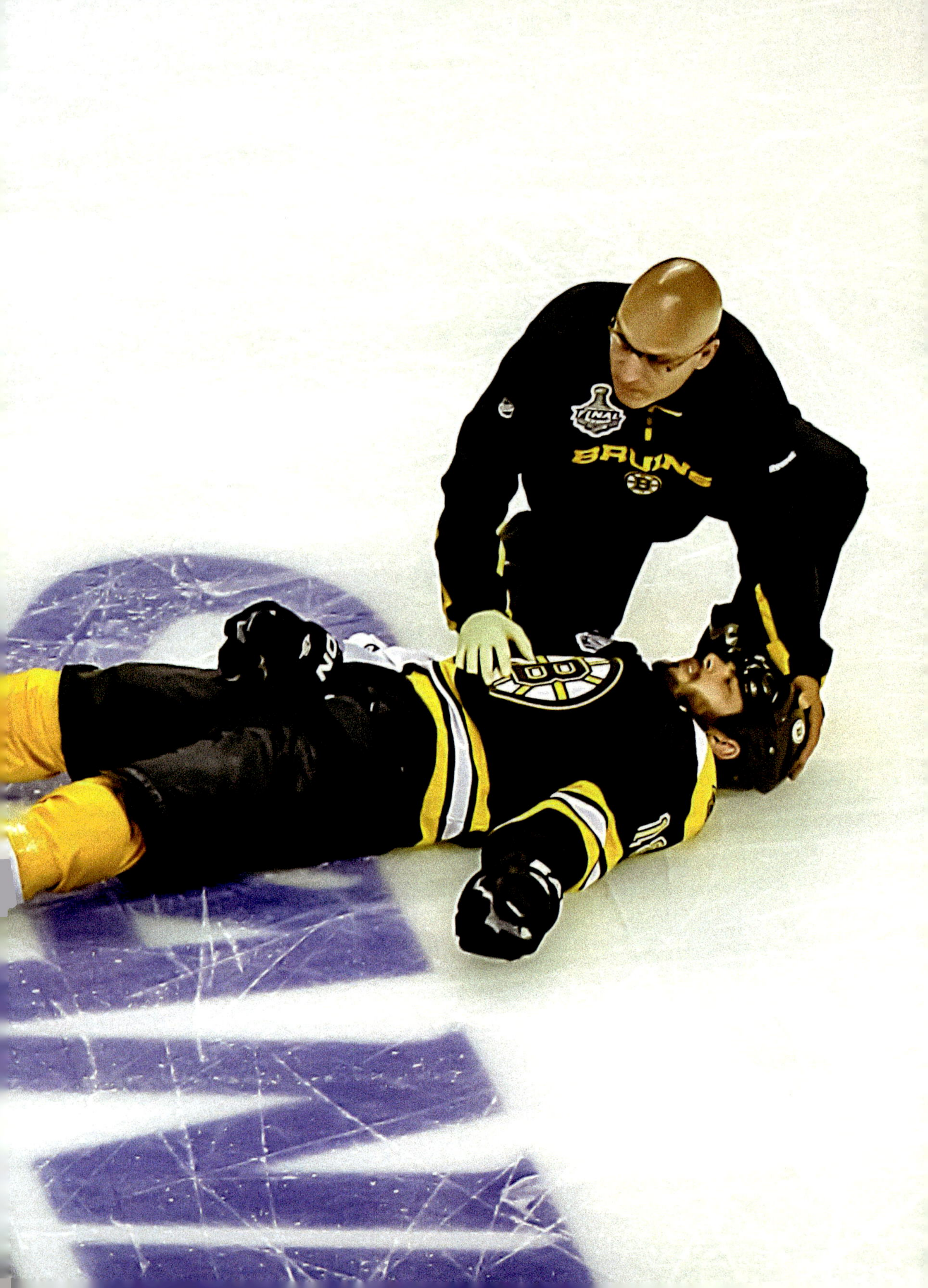
BRUINS

CHAPTER 1

WHAT IS A CONCUSSION?

Boston Bruins forward Nathan Horton streaked down the ice. The Bruins were facing the Vancouver Canucks in Game 3 of the 2011 Stanley Cup Final. Horton approached Vancouver's blue line and passed the puck to a teammate. But he went no farther. Canucks defenseman Aaron Rome slammed his shoulder into Horton's head. The blow knocked Horton off his feet. He landed headfirst on the ice.

Nathan Horton lies on the ice after a brutal hit to the head during the 2011 Stanley Cup Final.

For several minutes, Horton lay motionless as the medical staff took care of him. Soon, they carted him off on a stretcher and rushed him to the hospital. Horton had suffered a concussion.

A concussion is a type of brain injury. It occurs when the head moves back and forth quickly and violently. When that happens, the brain hits the inside of the skull. This impact damages the brain tissue. A concussion is typically caused by a blow to the head. However, it can also happen when a blow to the body jars the head.

Concussions can have several **symptoms**. They include headaches, confusion, and loss of memory. In addition, vision and hearing can weaken. Loss of balance is possible. And concussion victims often feel tired or sick.

Many sports involve actions that jar the head and body. As a result, the athletes who play these

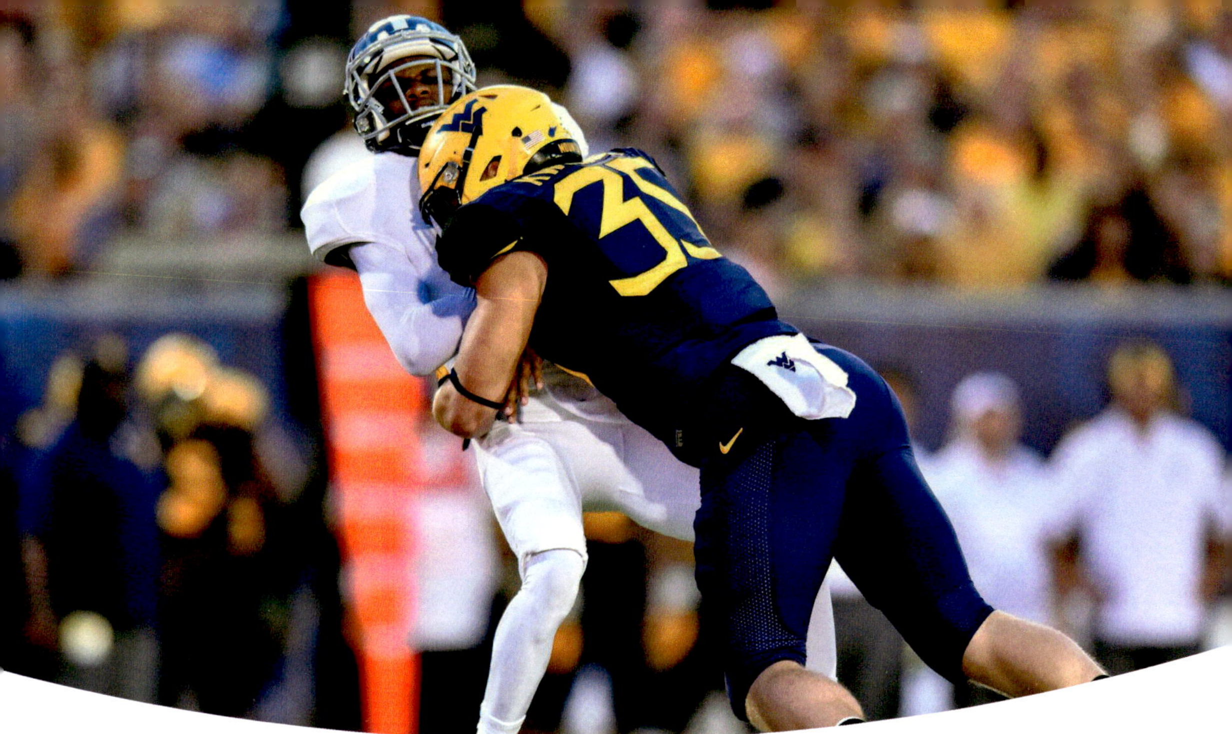

In terms of concussions, football is one of the most dangerous sports an athlete can play.

sports are at risk. In the past, athletes often continued playing after getting concussions. Players did not understand how serious these injuries were. But times have changed. The threat of brain damage has forced athletes to treat concussions with extreme care. Meanwhile, many sports leagues have created new rules to help athletes stay safe.

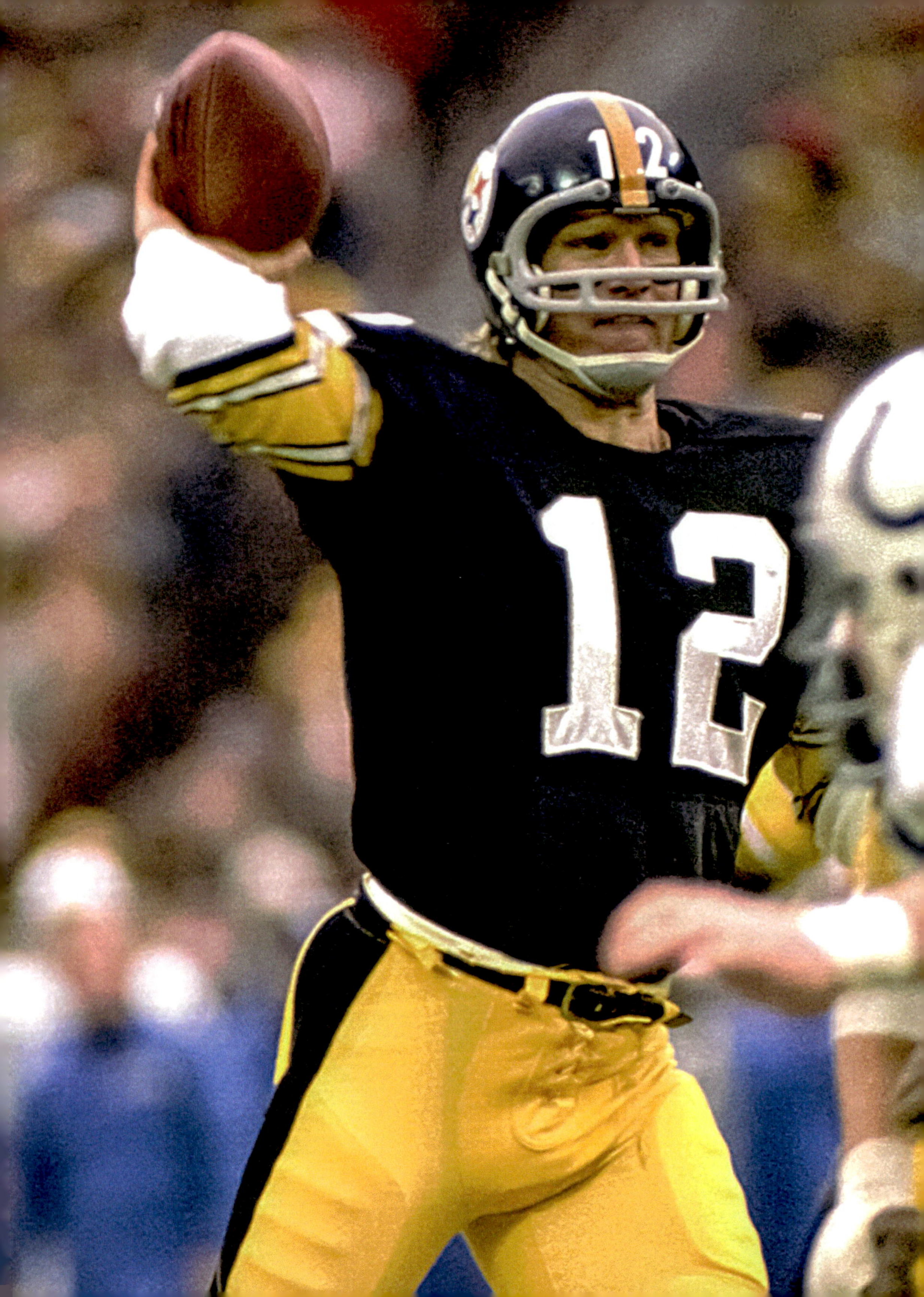
12
12

CHAPTER 2

AN ISSUE ONCE IGNORED

The National Football League (NFL) was founded in 1920. Since then, thousands of players have suffered head **trauma**. For decades, brutal hits to the head were an accepted part of the game. A prime example came in 1976. The Pittsburgh Steelers were taking on the Cleveland Browns. Steelers quarterback Terry Bradshaw dropped back to pass. Browns defensive end Joe Jones blasted through the line.

Due to concussions, Terry Bradshaw struggled with memory loss after his playing career ended.

Bradshaw had no chance to escape. Jones slammed the helpless quarterback on his head. Bradshaw fell unconscious. He was lucky his neck was not broken. But he lost all feeling in his body for two days. Jones received a 15-yard penalty for unnecessary roughness. However, he was not ejected from the game.

When a hit to the head occurred in decades past, the TV announcer might say the player had been "dinged." And when a player showed signs of dizziness, the announcer might say the player appeared to be "woozy." But in reality, these players were often dealing with concussions. And in many cases, the players remained in the game. That was simply the football mindset.

Football and hockey are often referred to as contact sports. But they are better defined as collision sports. In football, for example, linemen

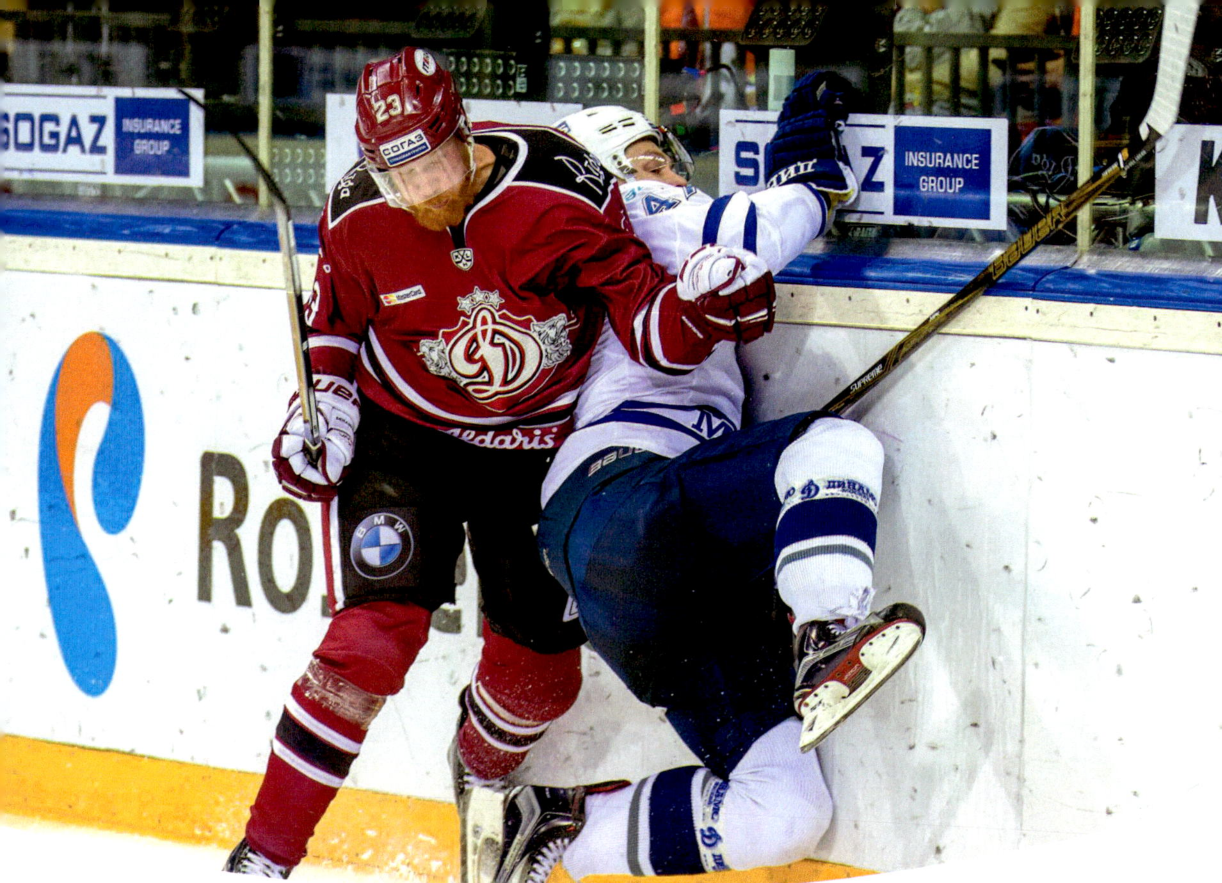

When a hockey player is checked, his or her brain can be slammed against the inside of the skull.

slam into one another on every play. Running backs, receivers, and quarterbacks can be victims of helmet-to-helmet hits. In hockey, players are often on the receiving end of high-speed **checks**. And players' heads can be jolted as they strike the ice. Any of these blows can cause concussions.

Repeated concussions can damage the brain's frontal lobe. This part of the brain is responsible for certain kinds of thinking. For this reason, athletes who suffer multiple concussions often deal with long-term health issues. Players may have problems with concentration, memory, and balance. They may also have trouble dealing with their emotions. These problems can continue after retirement. Over the long term, some players become depressed. Others become violent.

In the late 1990s and early 2000s, attitudes toward concussions slowly started to change. Retired and current athletes began speaking out. Also, medical studies showed more evidence of the problems concussions could lead to. Sports leagues, especially the NFL, faced increasing pressure to improve player safety. Leagues began creating new rules. Some required players to leave

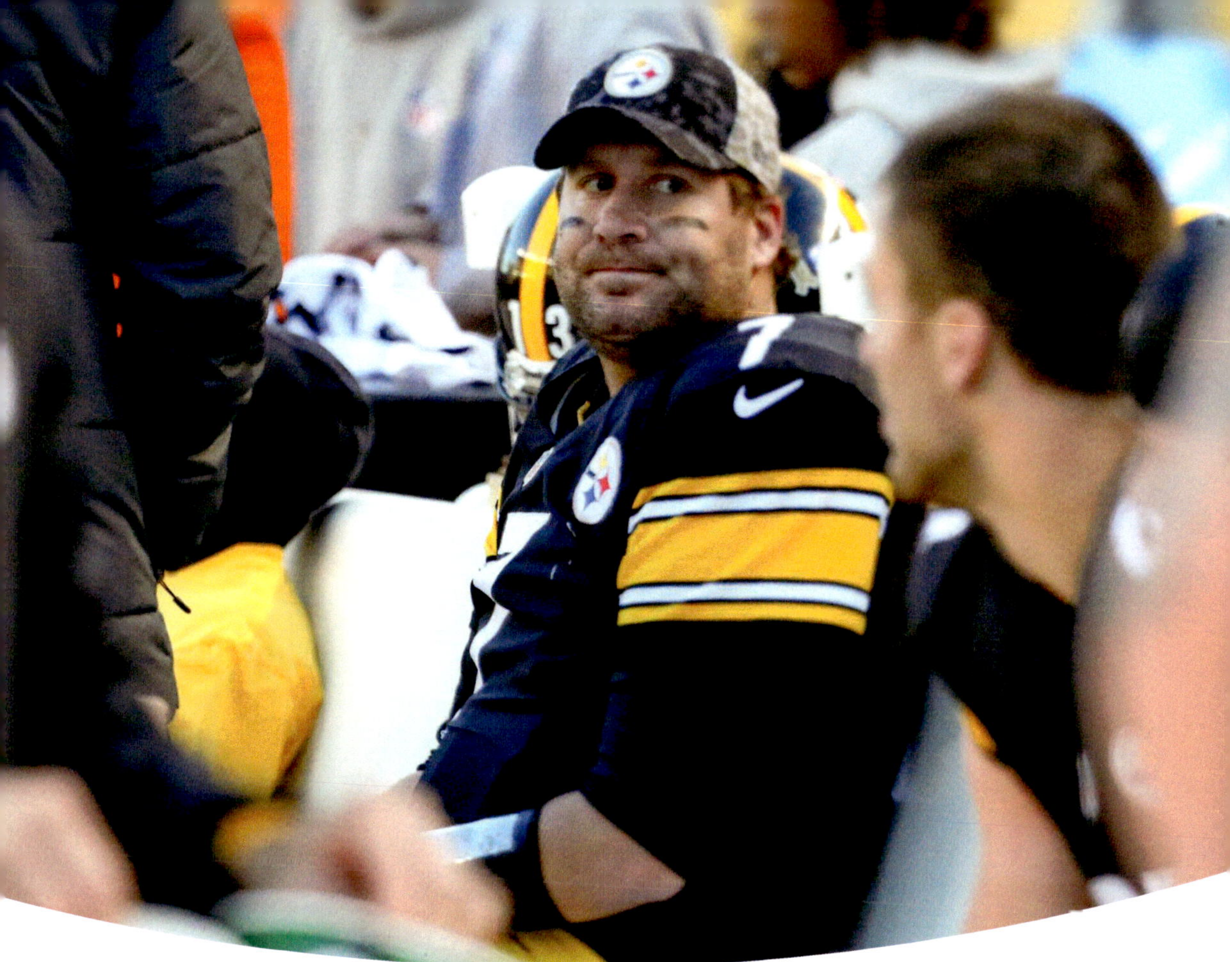

Steelers quarterback Ben Roethlisberger sits on the bench after a possible concussion during a 2015 game.

the game if they showed signs of concussions. Others required bigger penalties and fines to the players who delivered the hits. Leagues hoped to strike a balance between making players safer and keeping the action that fans love.

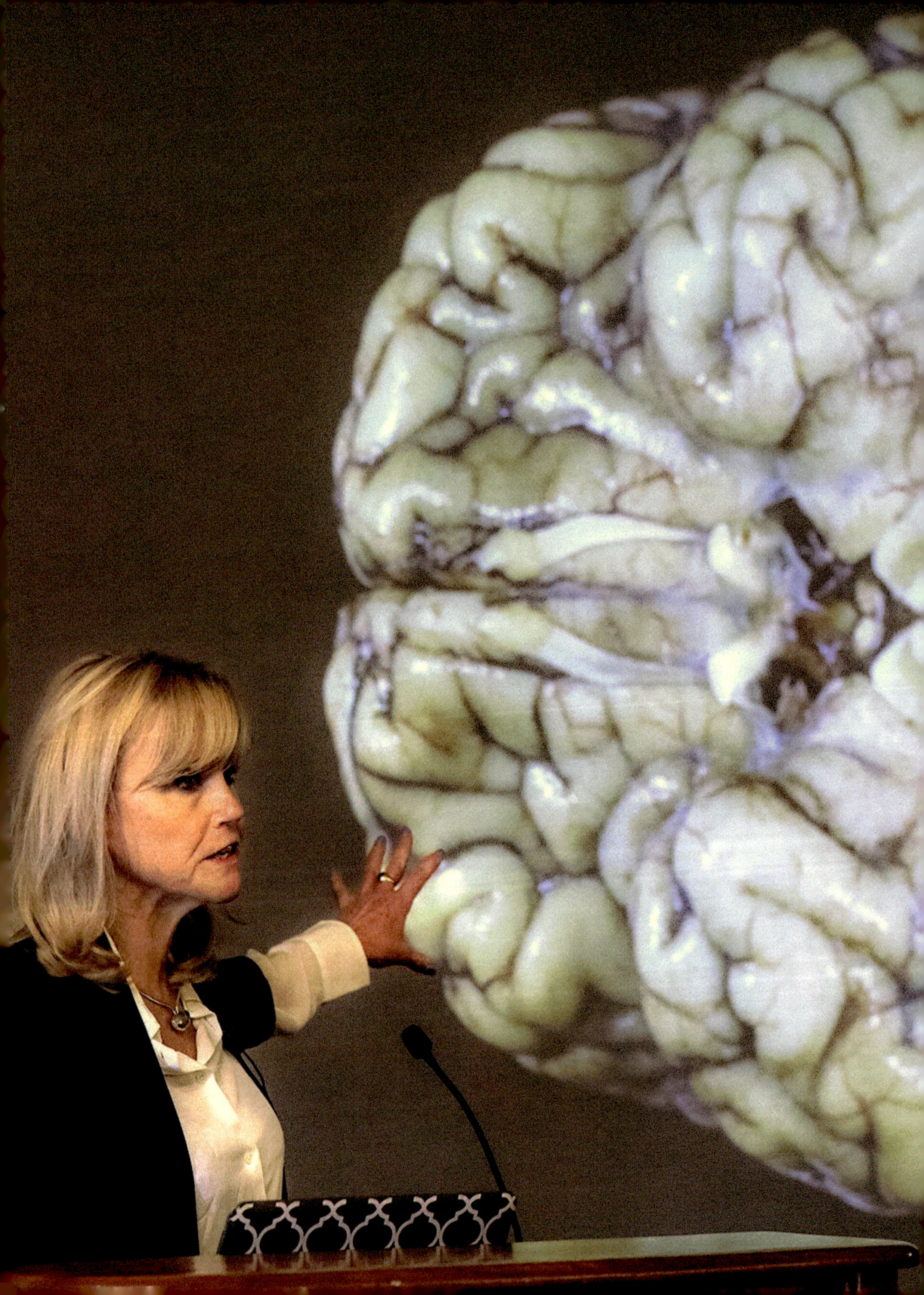

CHAPTER 3

LEGAL ACTION LEADS TO CHANGE

By the early 2000s, the issue of concussions could no longer be ignored. Medical studies proved that repeated head trauma could lead to **degenerative** brain disease. This type of disease causes the brain to become worse over time. People with the disease gradually lose the ability to speak and remember. They may also become violent or depressed.

A doctor discusses NFL player Aaron Hernandez, who suffered from degenerative brain disease. Hernandez was convicted of murder in 2015.

Former players suffering from this disease began complaining to the NFL. They believed the league had known about the dangers of concussions and kept this information a secret. They charged that the NFL did not want players to know that their mental and physical health was at risk every time they stepped onto the field.

Concussions in the NFL became a national issue. In 2009, the US government began an investigation. A doctor who worked for the NFL argued that the league was not at fault. He said there was no link between repeated concussions and permanent brain damage.

THINK ABOUT IT

Do you think the NFL ignored the issue of concussions before the 2000s? If so, what did the NFL have to gain by ignoring the issue?

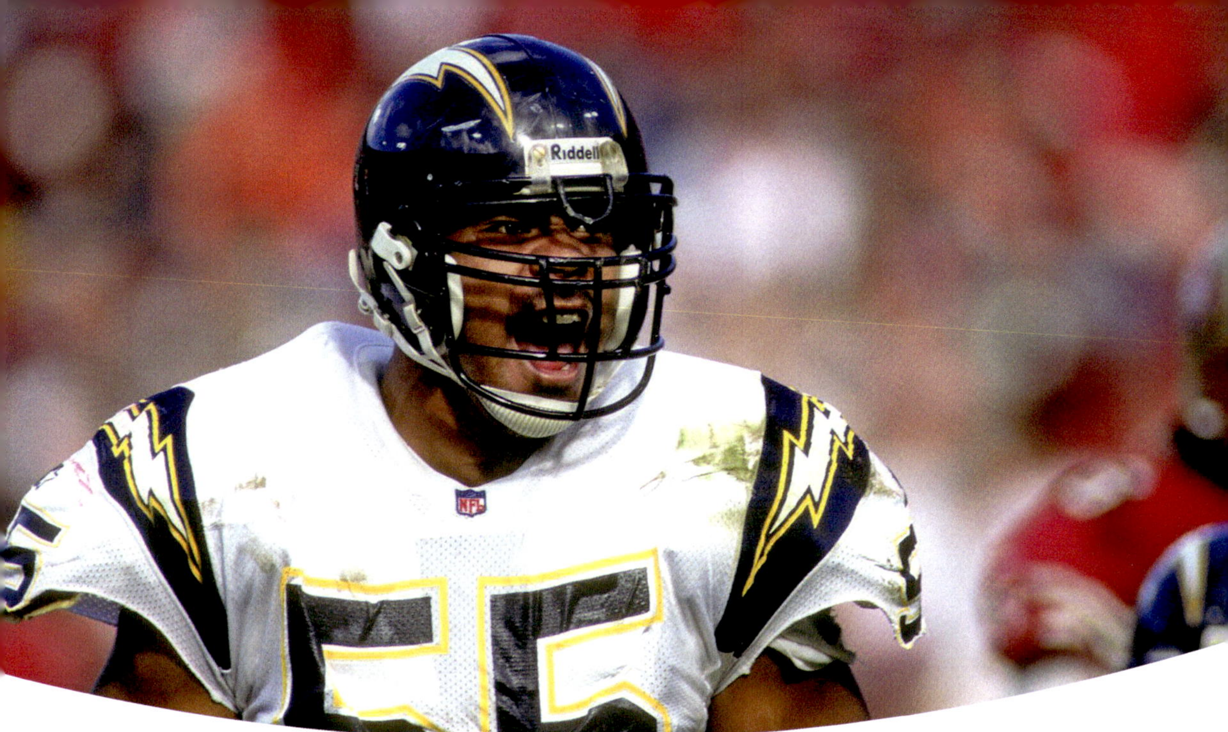

Hall of Fame linebacker Junior Seau took his own life in 2012. He suffered from degenerative brain disease.

Meanwhile, the stories of former players made news headlines. Several former players died by suicide. **Autopsies** showed clear evidence of long-term brain damage. In 2012, thousands of former players sued the NFL. The players claimed the league was **negligent**. They argued that the NFL had not told them about the link between concussions and permanent brain injury.

In 2013, the players agreed to accept an offer of $765 million from the NFL. That was an average of approximately $153,000 per player. However, a judge ruled that it was not enough money. In 2015, the court ordered the NFL to pay every player involved an average of $5 million.

In 2016, the NFL worked with players to create a concussion **protocol**. Any player who was suspected of being concussed would be removed from the game. Doctors would then examine the player. If he had concussion symptoms, he would not be allowed to return to the game. In fact, he could not play again until he was free of symptoms, even if that took weeks or months.

Referees got involved, too. They were instructed to call penalties on hits to the head, especially on hits against defenseless ballcarriers. Players who delivered violent hits could be ejected from games. They could even be suspended.

Several NFL players had already quit the sport in their prime rather than risk brain injury. The league and its players both understood the problem concussions were causing. And they were finally working together to create a solution.

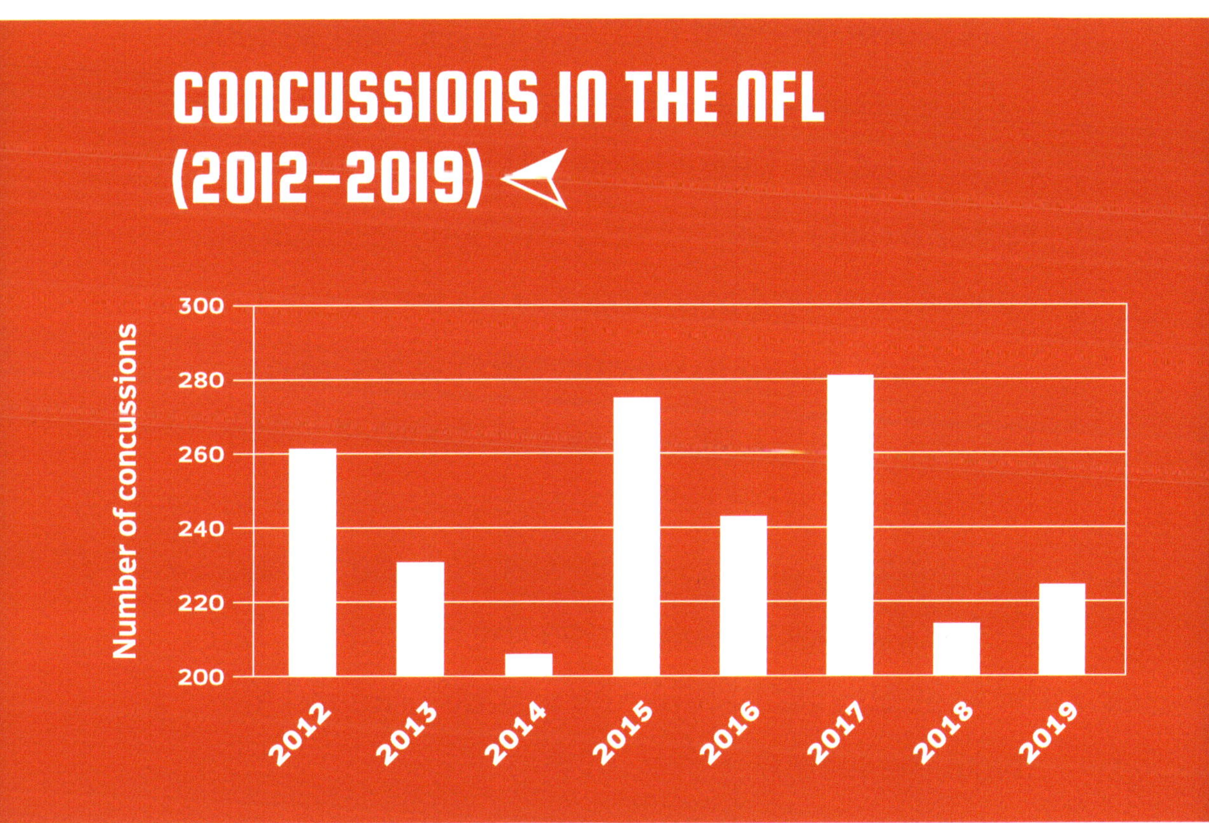

CHRIS BORLAND

Chris Borland seemed to be on the verge of stardom in 2014. The rookie linebacker led the San Francisco 49ers in tackles. He was also named to the NFL's all-rookie team. And he earned more than $1 million as a professional player.

However, Borland was worried. He had already suffered several concussions in his football career. He studied the threat to his long-term health. He realized there was a strong link between multiple concussions and permanent brain injury.

Borland talked to friends, teammates, and doctors. In 2015, he shocked the football world by announcing his retirement. Borland spoke to the media about his rookie year. He said he had suffered a concussion during the preseason. But he kept playing because he was determined to make the team.

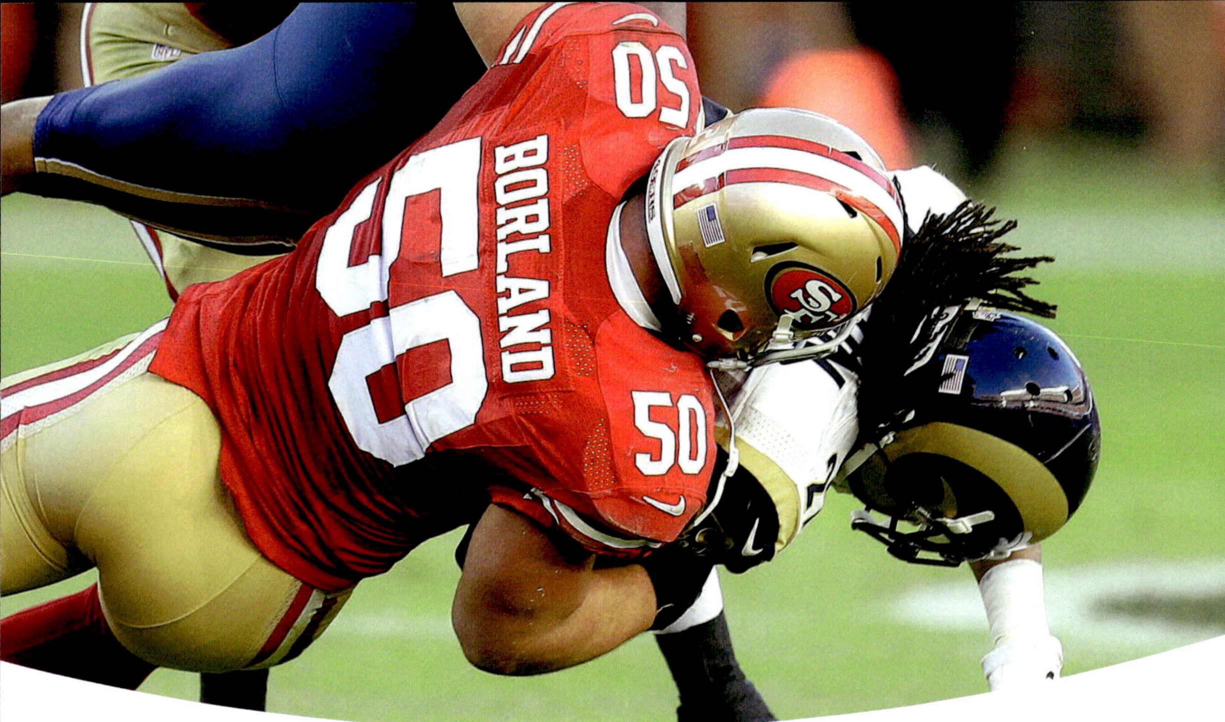

Chris Borland takes down the ballcarrier during his first and only NFL season.

Borland didn't think many people would pay attention to his retirement. Instead, he was targeted as a threat to the NFL. For instance, one sportswriter claimed Borland was a danger to the future of football. The writer believed that Borland's desire to avoid brain damage would convince young athletes to stop playing football. And that would impact the NFL by keeping talented players away.

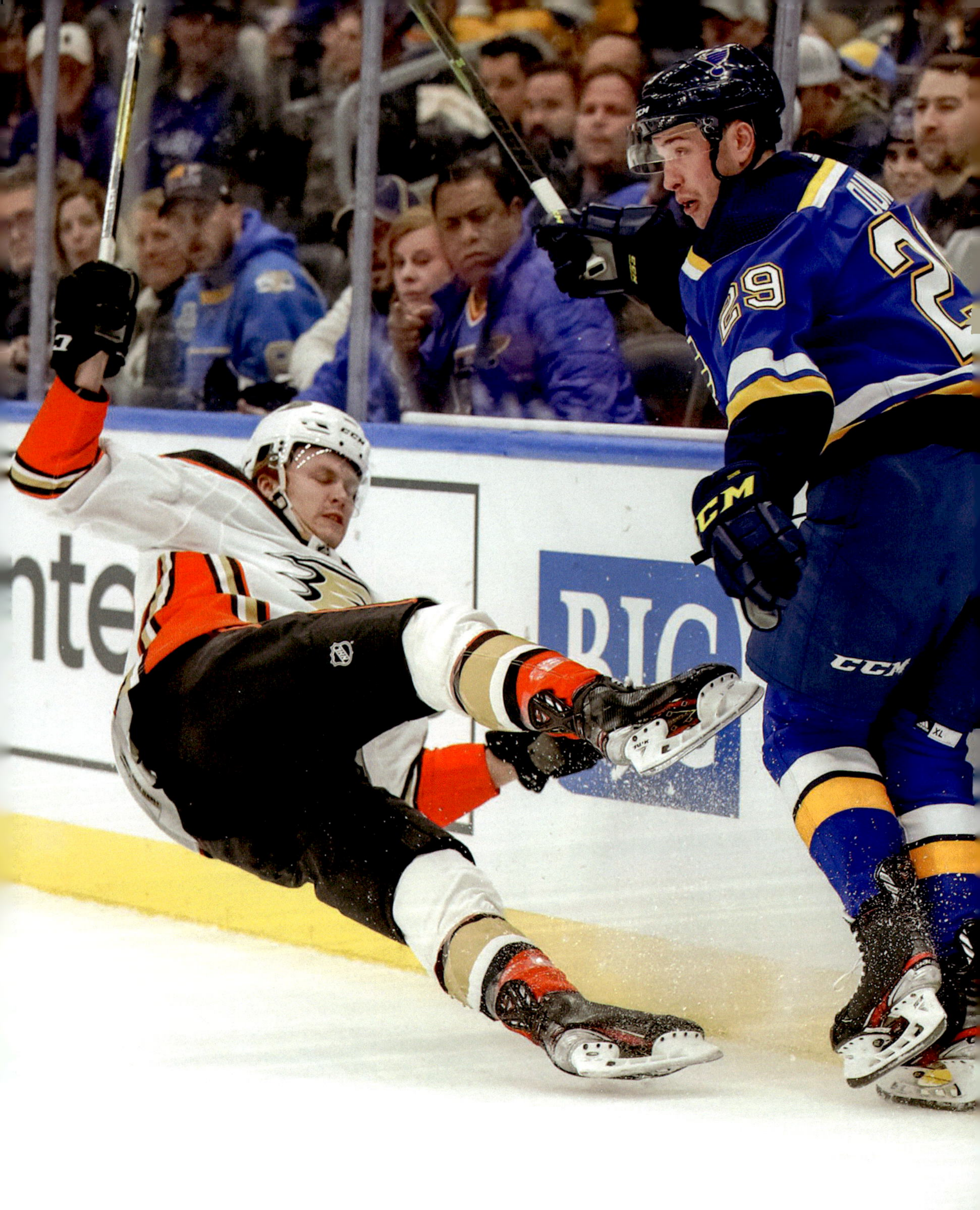
29
CCM
CCM

CHAPTER 4

OUTSIDE THE GRIDIRON

With all the attention the NFL receives, fans could easily assume that football is the only sport with a concussion problem. But studies suggest that hockey is just as dangerous. Many fans love hockey's fast pace and constant action. However, it can be a violent sport. Perhaps the most dangerous part of the game is checking. In the National Hockey League (NHL), players reach speeds of 20 miles per hour (32 km/h).

St. Louis Blues defenseman Vince Dunn knocks an opponent off his feet during a game in 2020.

When they slam opponents into the boards at high speeds, head injuries are a serious danger.

The NHL launched a concussion program in 1997. This program brought greater awareness to the problem of head injuries. It motivated teams to properly **diagnose** players who were suspected of being concussed.

In 2014, the league and players agreed to a new idea called the Player Safety Room. This room is at NHL headquarters in New York City. There, concussion experts watch each game. They keep an eye on any player who receives a hit to the head. They decide whether the player is showing signs of a concussion. If so, they can require the player to leave the game. In 2016, the NHL went a step further by creating a concussion protocol. A team must remove any player it believes could have suffered a head injury.

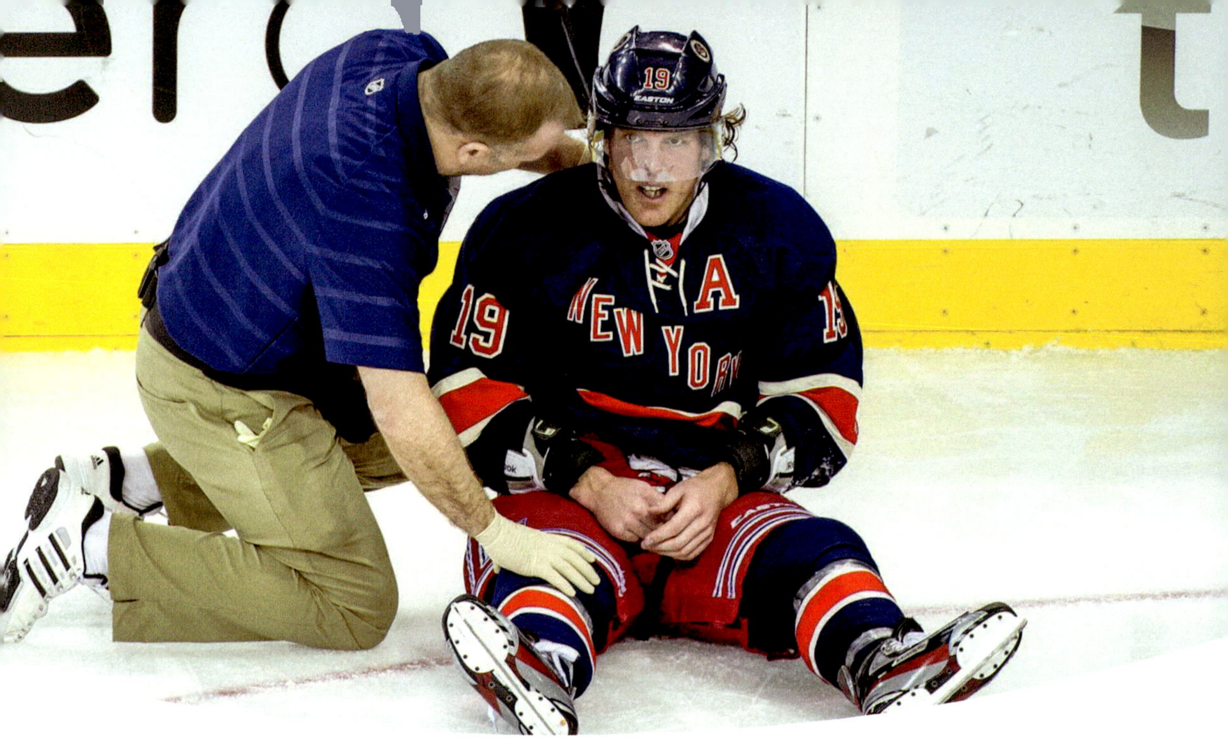

A trainer talks to New York Rangers center Brad Richards after an injury in 2013.

Hockey and football may carry the greatest risk of concussions. But other sports can be dangerous, too. Basketball was once thought of as a non-contact sport. However, modern training methods have made players in the National Basketball Association (NBA) stronger and faster than ever. Concussions can happen when players receive hard hits while driving to the hoop.

Other players may suffer blows to the head while battling for rebounds.

A concern for athlete safety motivated the NBA to launch a concussion policy in 2011. The protocol forces players to leave games when diagnosed with a concussion. They must stay on the sidelines until their symptoms are gone.

The NBA created very specific guidelines. A player cannot return to action until he is free of symptoms while resting. Then he must be checked by a team doctor. The player must prove that he can exert himself without symptoms. And the doctor must decide that the player is ready

THINK ABOUT IT

In your opinion, why didn't sports leagues create concussion protocols before the 1990s and 2000s?

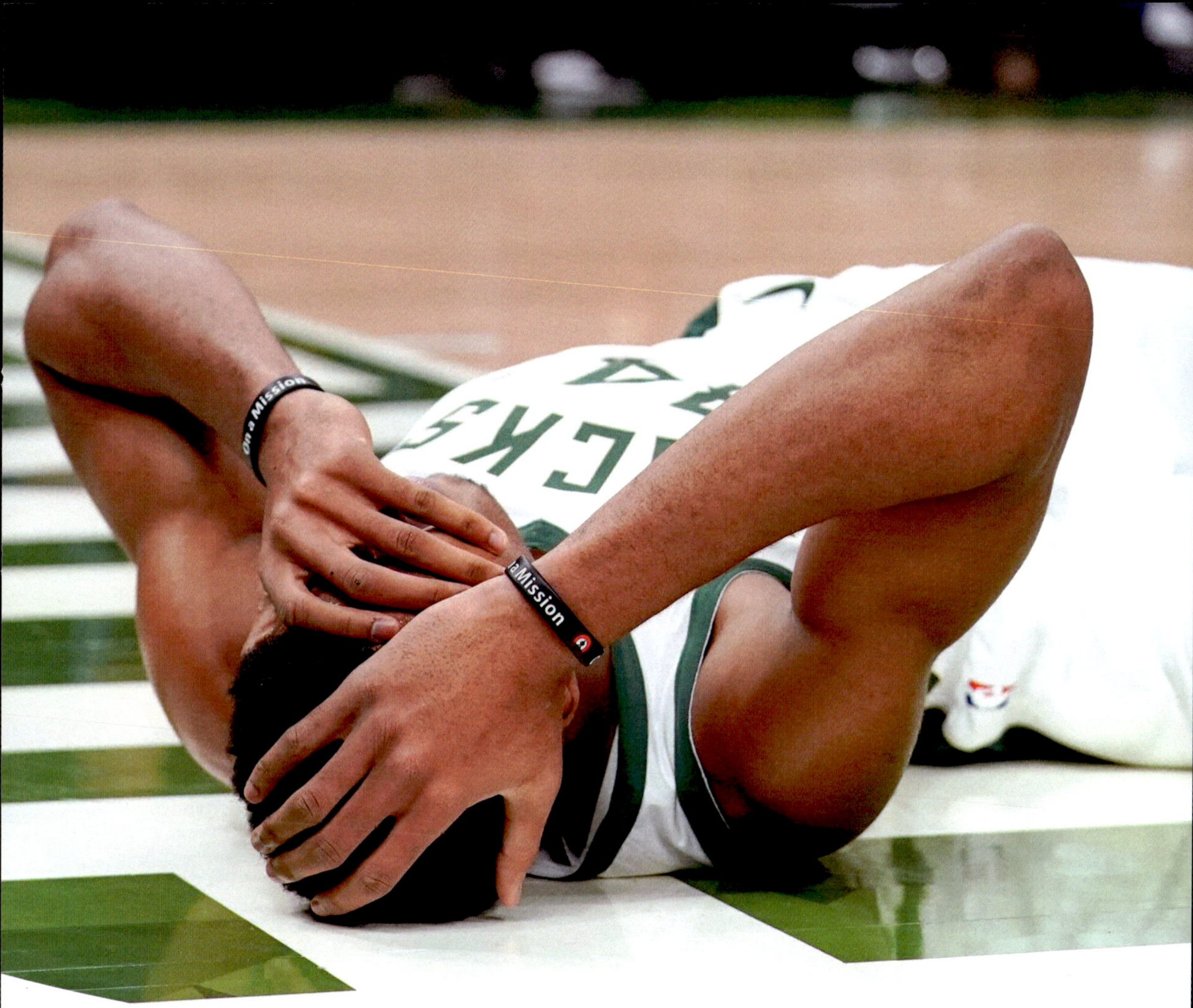

Milwaukee Bucks star Giannis Antetokounmpo missed a game in 2018 after suffering a concussion.

to return. In addition, the doctor must discuss that decision with the director of the league's concussion program. However, the final decision rests with the team doctor.

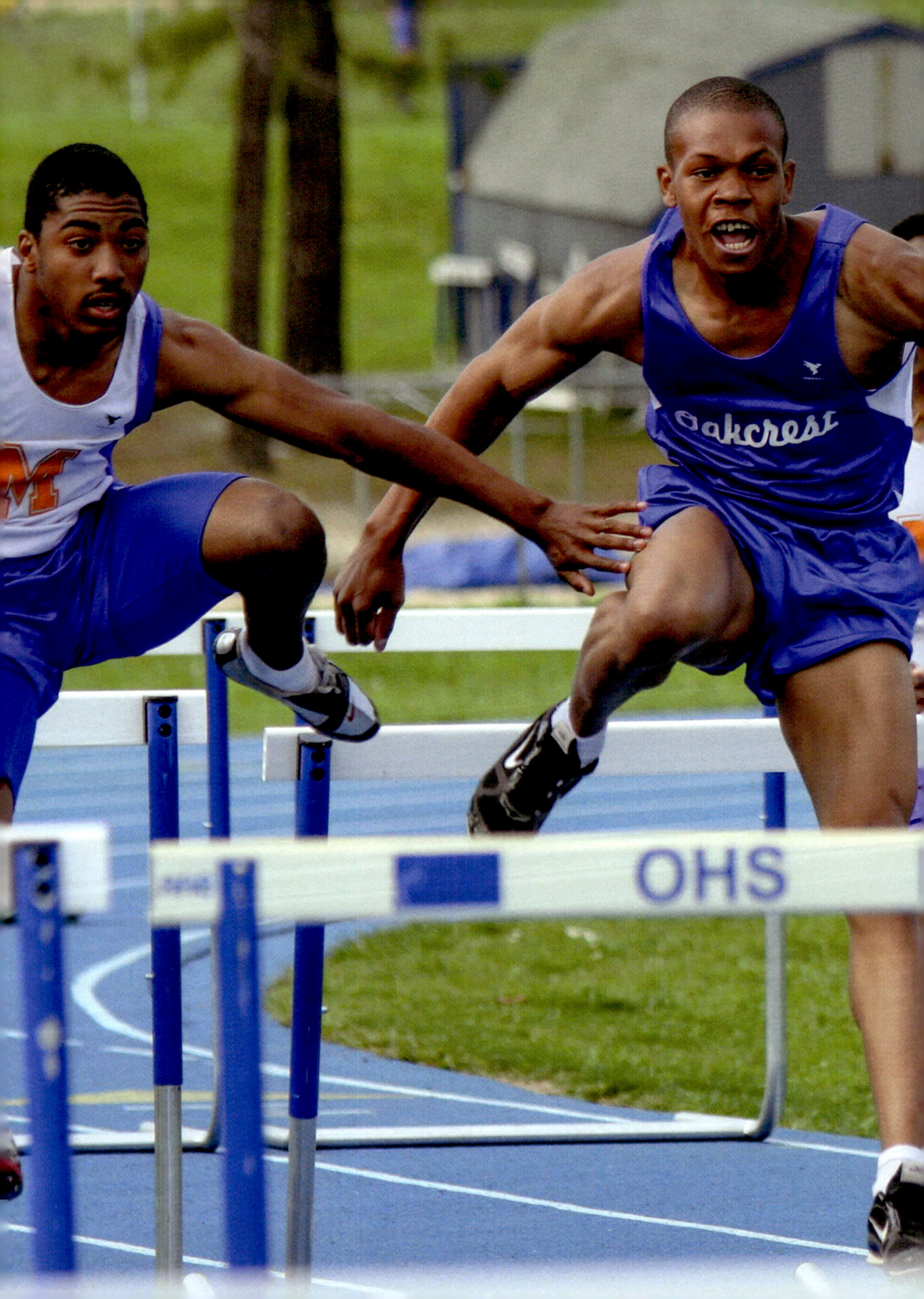
Oakcrest
OHS

CHAPTER 5

A DANGER TO YOUNG PLAYERS

Concussion victims are not limited to pro athletes. Players at the youth level face the danger of concussions as well. The odds of getting a concussion depend on the amount of contact in the sport. Concussions are far more common in hockey than in tennis, for example. Gender can also be a factor. Girls tend to suffer more head injuries than boys when playing soccer and basketball. Researchers are not sure why.

In terms of concussion risk, track is a safer sport than football.

They think one possible reason is that girls tend to have weaker neck muscles. As a result, girls' heads move more when they are hit.

Of course, no sport is without risk. But of all the sports that young athletes play, football is the one that results in the most concussions. This danger has led many young players to quit football. In addition, some parents have forced their children to choose safer sports. That's because parents and young athletes have started to gain a better understanding of the risk factors for concussions. A risk factor is anything that increases a person's chances of getting an injury. When it comes to concussions, the biggest risk factor is prior head injuries.

Parents and young athletes take risk factors seriously. After all, a single concussion can lead to headaches, anxiety, and even learning disabilities.

And multiple concussions can do even more serious, long-lasting damage.

Most doctors believe education is the best way to reduce concussions. They say young athletes should learn about the most effective ways to stay safe. One way is to do exercises that strengthen the neck. This can improve the ability to absorb blows that would otherwise impact the brain.

HIGH SCHOOL SPORTS WITH THE HIGHEST CONCUSSION RATES

This graph shows the number of concussions per 10,000 athlete exposures. An athlete exposure is when a player takes part in a game or practice. So, if 25 players attend a practice, there are 25 athlete exposures.

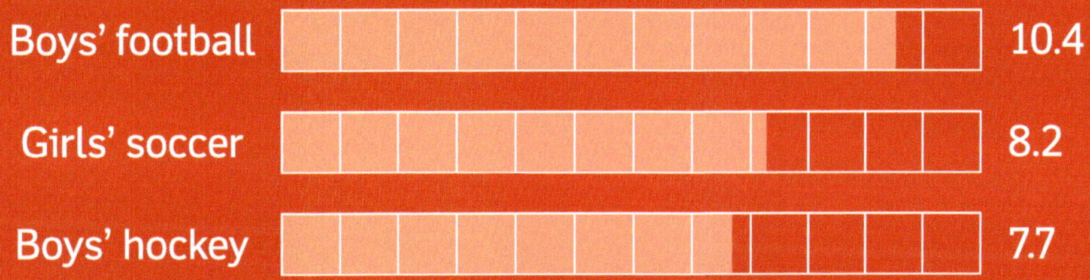

Sport	Rate
Boys' football	10.4
Girls' soccer	8.2
Boys' hockey	7.7

Another way to improve safety is to use tackling methods that don't impact the head. The tackler should keep his or her head to the side while driving a shoulder into the runner's chest or thigh.

Helmets and other protective equipment can also help guard against head injuries. But studies show that safety gear reduces concussions by only 20 percent. Many parents and athletes say that isn't good enough. For this reason, football **participation** levels have continued to drop.

The number of boys playing high school football peaked in 2009. By 2019, the number had fallen by nearly 10 percent. Even football-crazed Texas has seen a decline in participation. In 2016,

THINK ABOUT IT

Suppose you were deciding whether to play high school football. What factors would you consider?

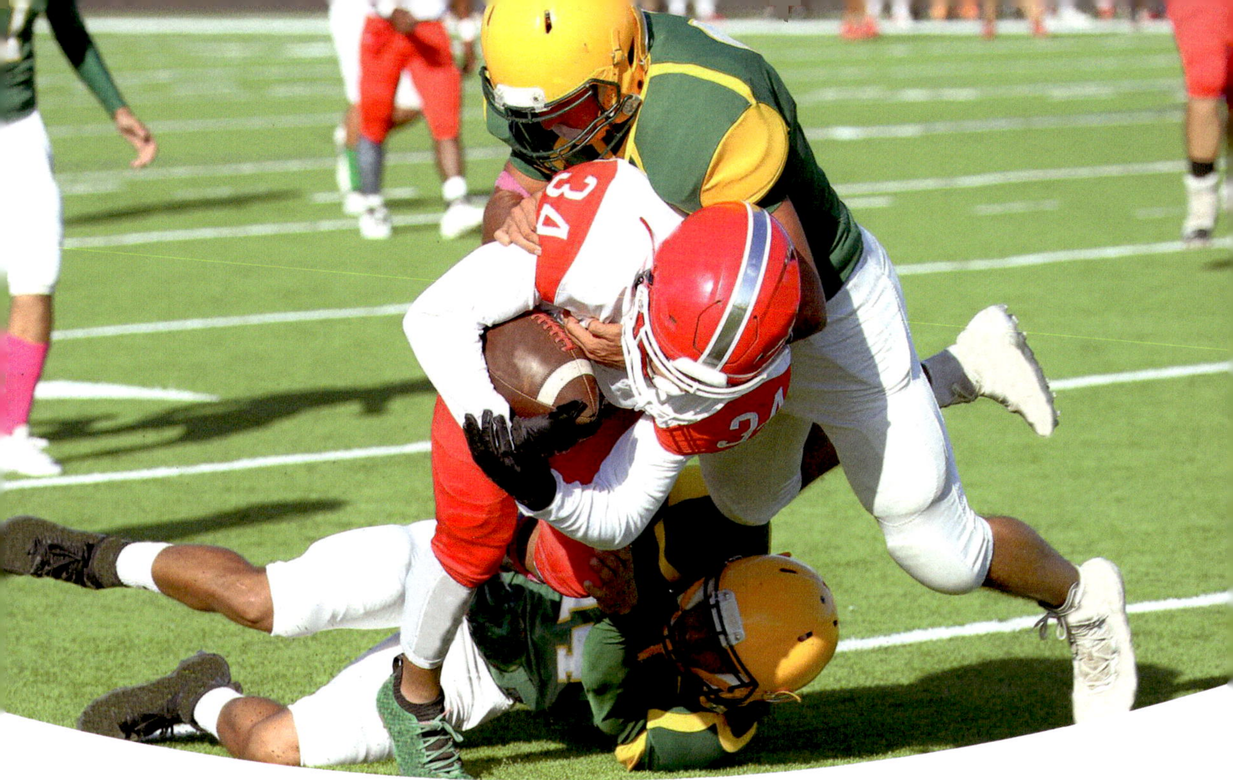

Using tackling methods that don't impact the head is one of the keys to preventing concussions.

the state averaged 153 football players per high school. By 2018, the number had fallen to 125.

Despite these declines, football remains the most popular sport at the youth level. And most experts believe it will remain popular for many years to come. Still, there is concern for the game's future. Players and parents worry about concussions leading to permanent brain damage.

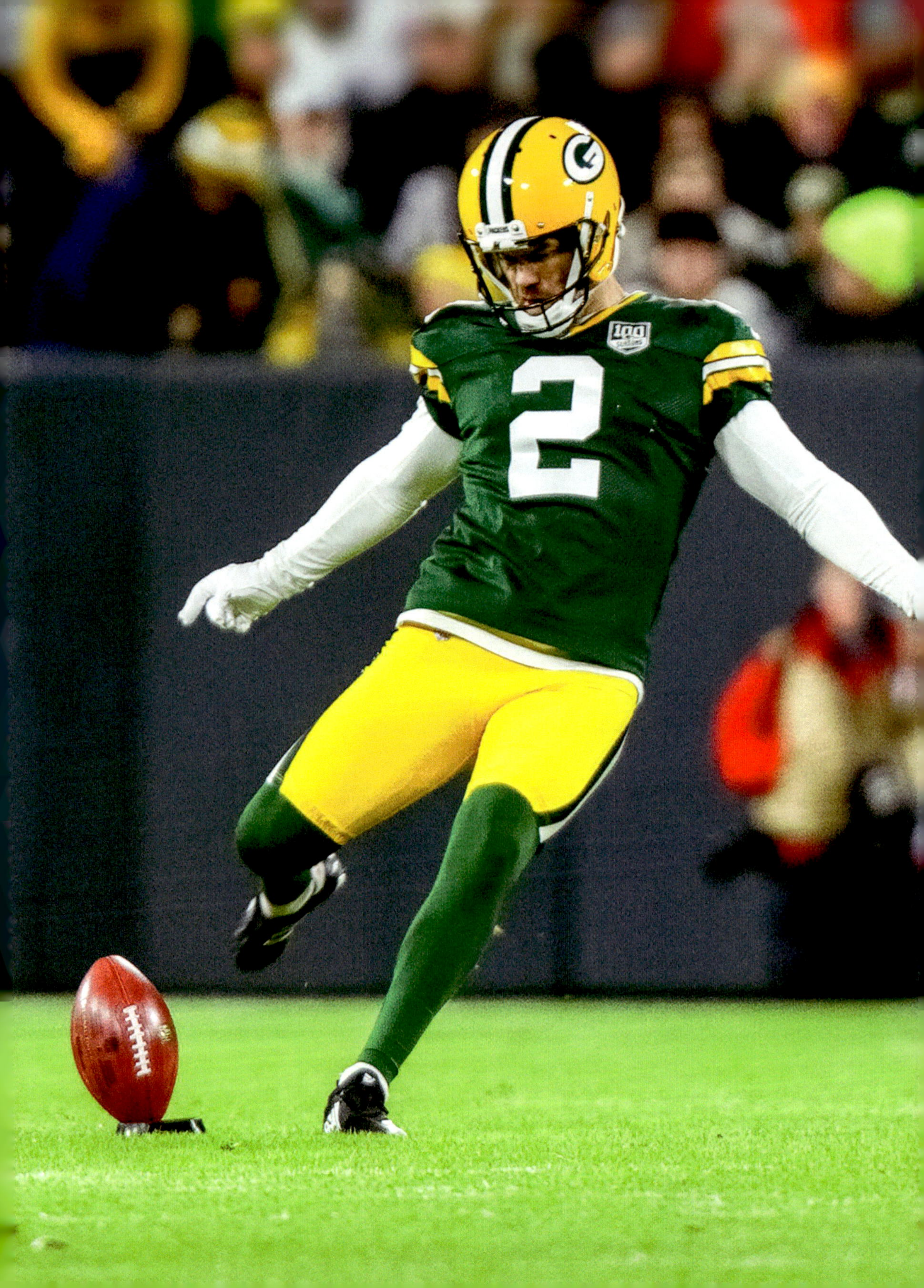
2

CHAPTER 6

SEARCHING FOR SOLUTIONS

For most NFL fans, it would be hard to imagine watching flag football on Sundays. But banning tackling would be the only sure way to end the risk of concussions. The NFL is not about to go that far. However, the league has created new rules to increase safety. For instance, kickoff returns are one of the most dangerous parts of the game. On this play, players run down the field at full speed and then crash into one another.

In the 2019 NFL season, more than 60 percent of kickoffs were not returned.

Not surprisingly, kickoffs have resulted in a high rate of head injuries over the years.

In response, the NFL came up with a plan that would limit the number of kickoff returns. For many years, kickoffs had taken place at the 30-yard line. But in 2011, the league moved kickoffs to the 35-yard line. Kickers were now five yards closer. As a result, they booted more kickoffs into the end zone. In many cases, the ball was impossible to return. That meant the play resulted in a touchback. The receiving team took over at the 20-yard line.

In 2010, before the new rule took effect, the NFL recorded 35 concussions on kickoffs. In 2011, the number dropped to 20. The experiment had worked. But there was still room for improvement.

In 2016, the NFL changed its touchback rule. The receiving team would now get the ball at

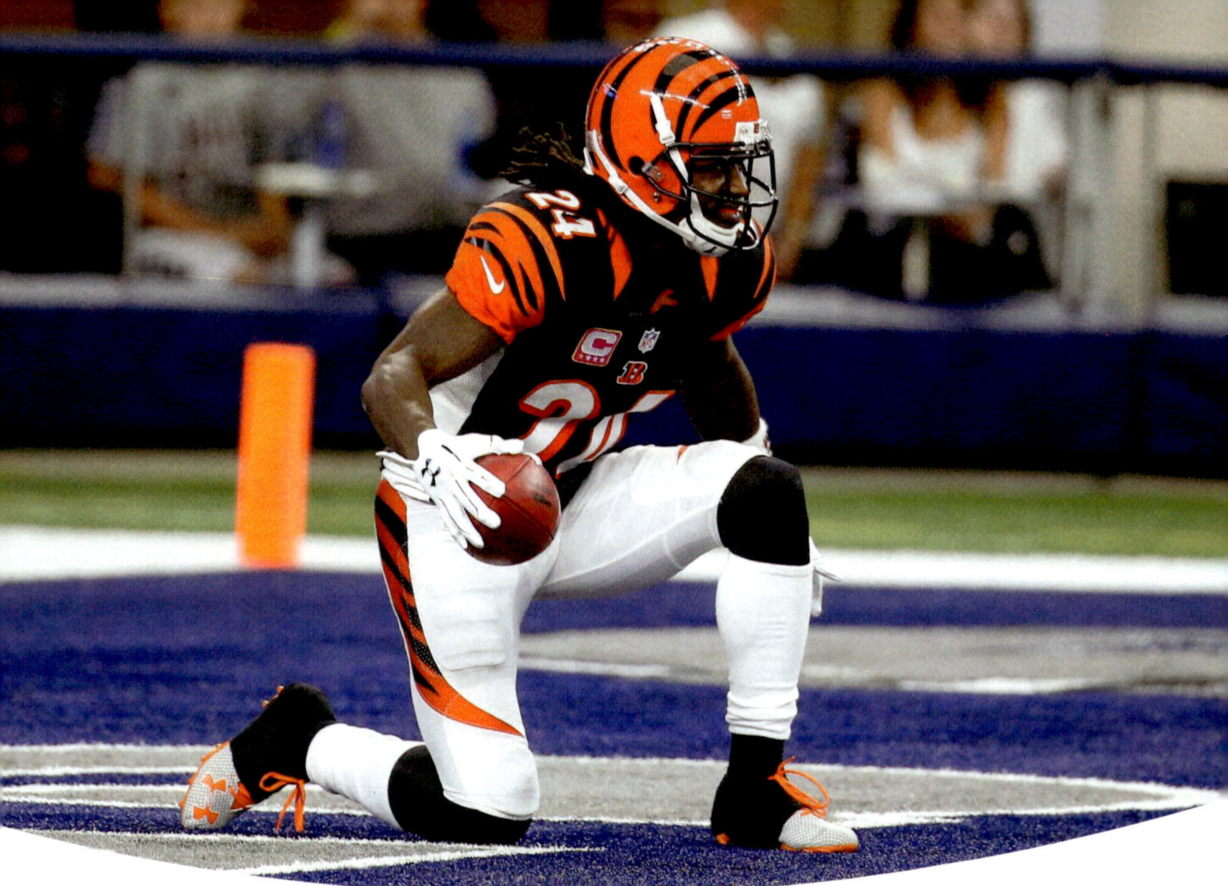

A decrease in kickoff returns has led to a decrease in concussions.

the 25-yard line instead of the 20-yard line. This change gave teams an even bigger reason to avoid returning kickoffs.

Leagues at other levels took these changes even further. In college football, one **conference** moved kickoffs up to the 40-yard line in 2016.

The previous year, 21 percent of all concussions had happened on kickoffs, even though kickoffs made up only 6 percent of all plays. Thanks to the change, concussion rates dropped by 68 percent in 2016.

Another way that football teams are reducing head injuries is by limiting tackling in practice. A study of high school athletes showed that limiting or banning tackling during practice reduced the number of concussions.

Timothy A. McGuine was one of the scientists who ran the study. Despite the study's results, McGuine did not support banning tackling during games. He believed the benefits of competing outweighed the risks involved.

Still, McGuine did have advice for parents and high school athletes. He urged people to be aware of the dangers of multiple concussions. He warned

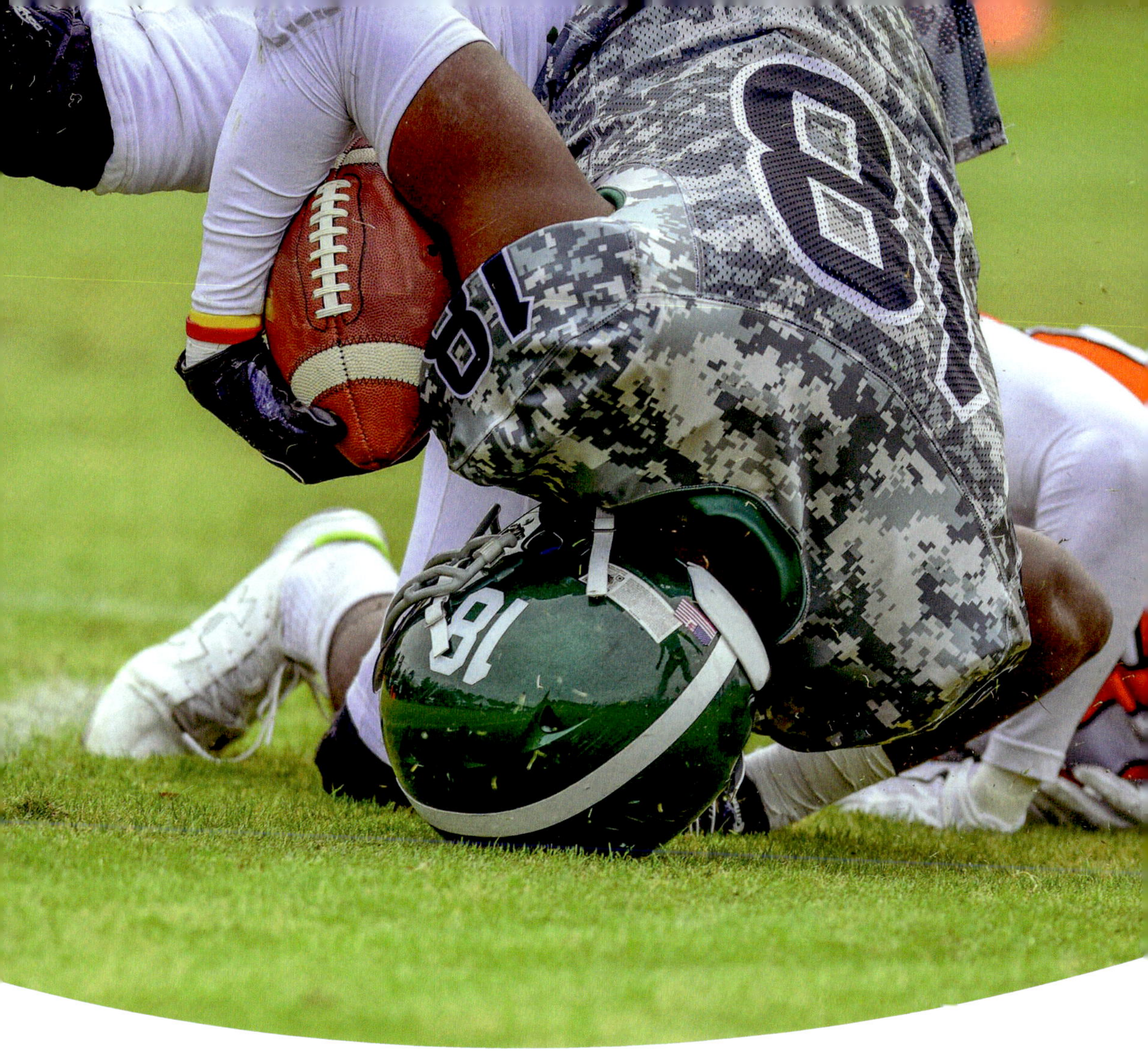

Many athletes choose to play football despite knowing the risks.

that any player who has sustained one concussion is at greater risk for another. Choosing whether to keep playing can be a difficult decision.

FOOTBALL HELMETS

Football helmets were made of leather until the late 1930s. By the 1940s, most helmets were made of hard plastic. Foam inside the helmet was designed to cushion the player's head.

Over the years, engineers have continued working to improve helmets. They test dozens of different models. These tests help engineers figure out which designs are safest.

In 2019, the NFL declared that helmets with foam padding would no longer be allowed. Instead, the padding must be made from a specific type of plastic. Some players did not like the new models. They said the old helmets were more comfortable. Even so, studies proved that the new helmets offered greater protection.

Scientists point out that helmets are designed to protect athletes from skull fractures, not concussions. Even the most high-tech helmet

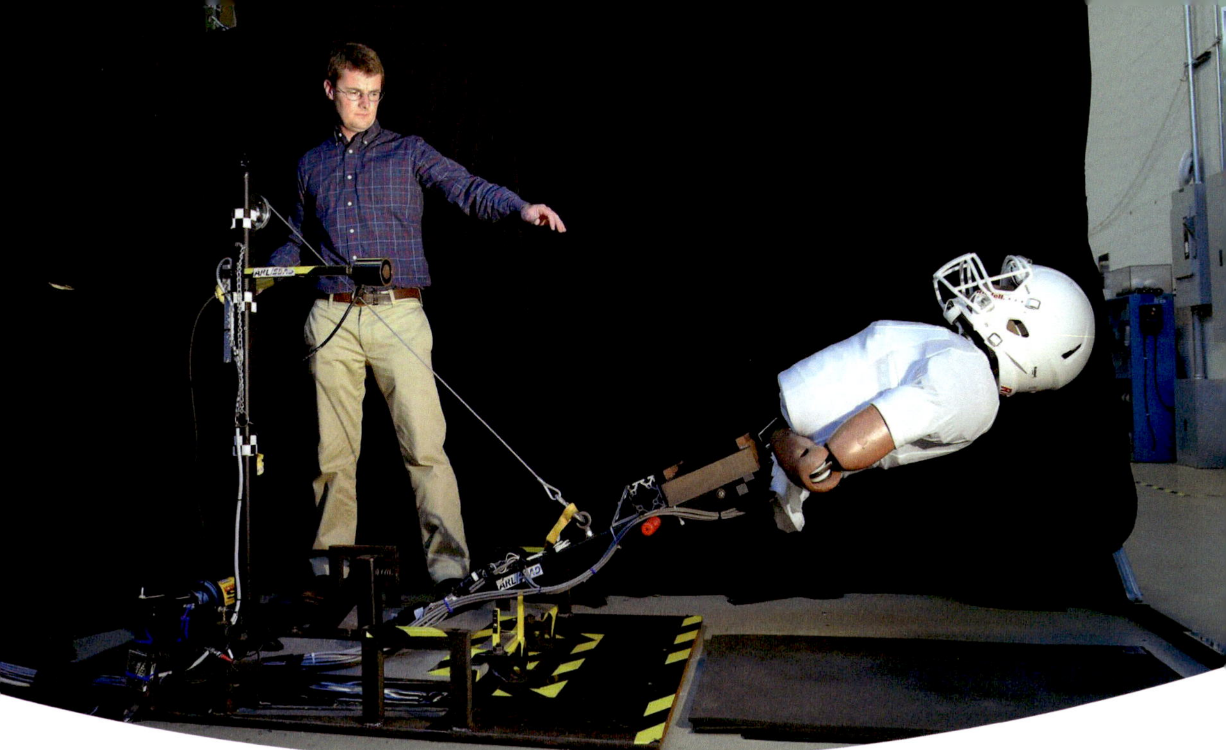

A researcher uses a dummy to test a football helmet.

cannot stop the brain from moving inside the skull. And that is what causes a concussion. In fact, one study showed that modern helmets are no safer than leather helmets when it comes to protecting athletes from concussions.

According to scientists, helmets are only part of the solution. They say rule changes are a much more effective way to keep players safe. Players must also be taught to avoid hits to the head.

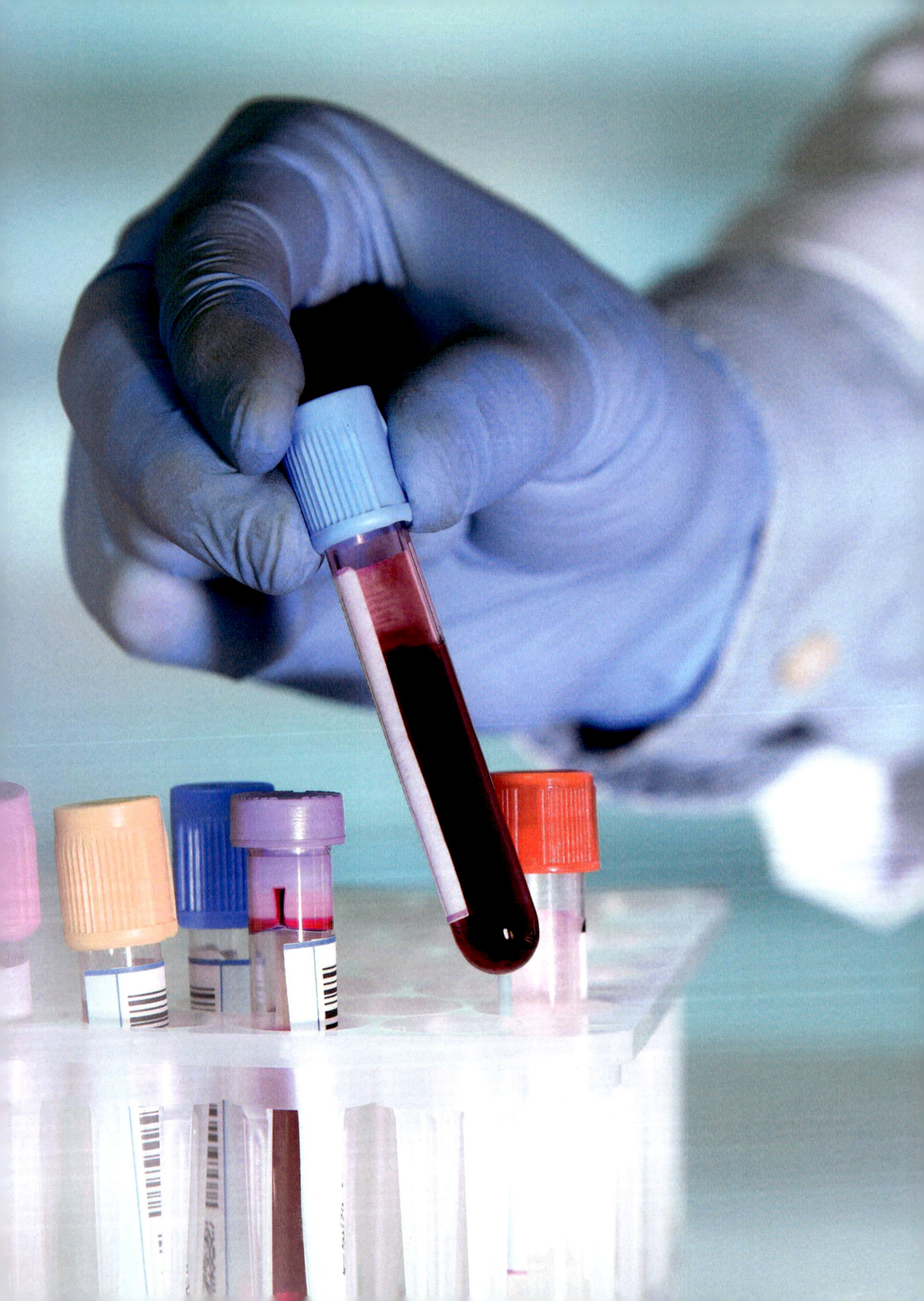

CHAPTER 7

HOPE FOR THE FUTURE

Researchers hope to prevent, detect, and treat concussions. They have worked on a variety of new technologies. One of their discoveries was that blood tests can diagnose head injuries. Researchers found two **proteins** in the blood that show up at higher levels after an athlete is concussed. Scientists then figured out how much of each protein is too much. If an athlete has more than that level, he or she likely has a concussion.

Blood tests are approximately 97 percent effective in identifying damaged brain tissue.

At the University of Pennsylvania, scientists developed a material that changes the color of a helmet upon impact. The helmet turns from red to green when struck lightly. But it turns purple when hit harder. The color indicates whether a player needs to be checked for a concussion.

At Harvard University, scientists are working on a pill that could help athletes who have suffered multiple head injuries. The pill would help slow the spread of degenerative brain disease. This disease is common among people who have sustained multiple concussions.

Dartmouth University football coach Buddy Teevens has worked to prevent concussions during practice. Teevens uses a mobile tackling dummy. The remote-controlled dummy allows players to practice tackling with proper form. That way, players can avoid head impact.

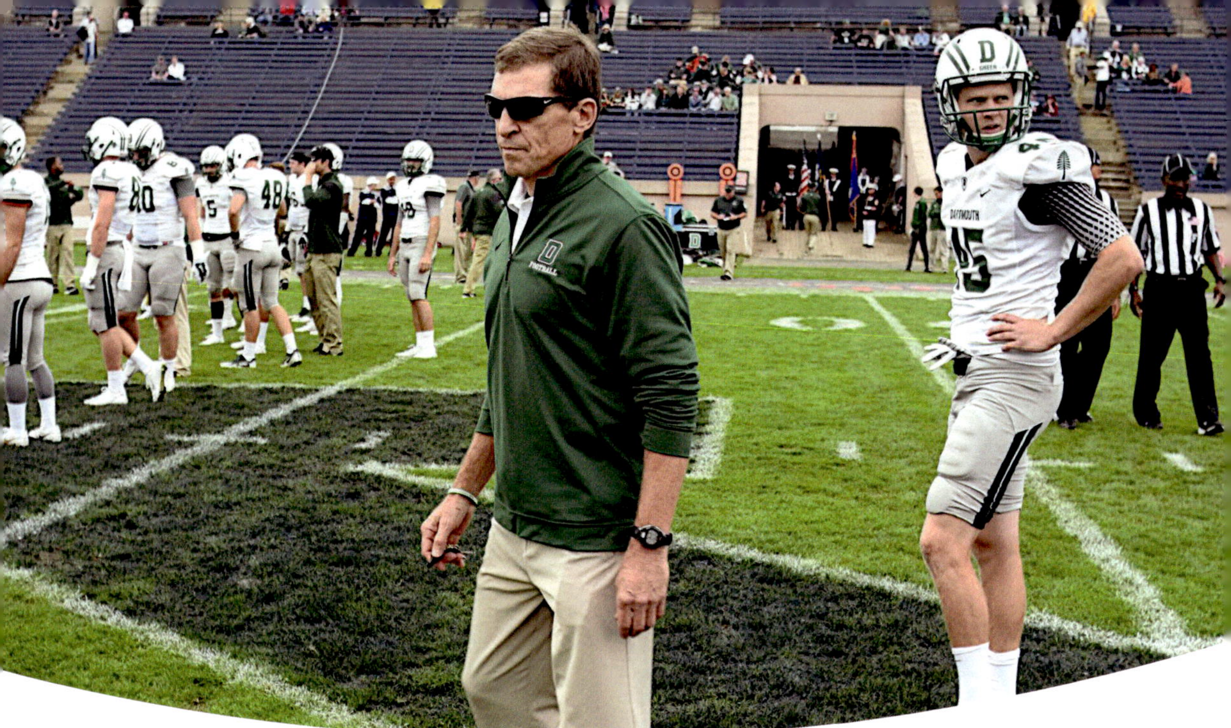

Buddy Teevens helps his team warm up before a 2016 game.

Researchers are not trying to remove all contact from sports. They simply want to keep athletes healthier during and after their careers. With further research, education, and rule changes, players will be in a better position to avoid concussions. That way, players can stay healthier while taking part in the action that fans love.

FOCUS ON
CONCUSSIONS

Write your answers on a separate piece of paper.

1. Write a letter to a friend explaining the main ideas of Chapter 5.
2. Do you believe sports leagues have done enough to reduce the number of concussions? Why or why not?
3. Other than football, which professional sport has the highest rate of concussions?
   - A. tennis
   - B. basketball
   - C. hockey
4. To reduce the number of concussions in football, why might changing the rules be more effective than improving helmets?
   - A. because not all football players are required to wear helmets
   - B. because helmets can't stop a player's brain from hitting the skull
   - C. because changing the rules would be less expensive

Answer key on page 48.

GLOSSARY

autopsies
Medical examinations to figure out the cause of death.

checks
Hits in which hockey players slam their bodies into opposing players.

conference
A group of teams within a league.

degenerative
Causing loss of physical or mental strength, often related to age or injury.

diagnose
To identify an illness or disease.

negligent
Failing to be careful.

participation
The act of taking part in something.

proteins
Molecules that are important in telling a living cell what to do.

protocol
A specific set of rules that are followed.

symptoms
Signs of an illness or disease.

trauma
An injury caused by a hard hit.

TO LEARN MORE

BOOKS

Abramovitz, Melissa. *Brain Science*. Minneapolis: Abdo Publishing, 2016.

Goldsmith, Connie. *Traumatic Brain Injury: From Concussion to Coma*. Minneapolis: Lerner Publications, 2014.

Rose, Simon. *Heads Up! Concussion Awareness*. New York: Crabtree Publishing, 2018.

NOTE TO EDUCATORS

Visit **www.focusreaders.com** to find lesson plans, activities, links, and other resources related to this title.

INDEX

Answer Key: 1. Answers will vary; **2.** Answers will vary; **3.** C; **4.** B